Published By Nicholas Thompson

@ Sherry Fowler

Low Carb: Benefits and Recipes of to Weight Loss

Through Carbohydrate Management

All Right RESERVED

ISBN 978-1-7782903-0-5

TABLE OF CONTENTS

Beef Goulash 1

Upside Down Breakfast Soufflé 3

Low Carb Pancake Crepes 5

Baby Spinach Omelet 7

Ground Beef With Sliced Bell Peppers 9

Garlic Lime Chicken Fajitas 11

Protein Waffles 13

The Amazing Low Carb Goulash (Hungarian Stew) Recipe 14

Vanilla-Pumpkin Protein Smoothie 16

Orangey Apple-Veggie Drink 17

Low-Carb Mashed Cauliflower 18

Low-Carb Chicken And Mushroom Soup 19

White Bread 21

Peach And Sour Cream Muffins 23

The Coconut Macadamia Bars 25

Low Carb, Paleo, Grain-Free Flax Waffles 27

Broccoli Cheddar Soup 29

Onion Soup 30

Coconut White Chocolate Fudge 32

Coffee Cake Cinnamon Collagen Fat Bombs 34

Scrambled Eggs With Bacon And Chard 35

Avocado Chicken Omelet 37

Cheese Chive Waffles 39

Tex Mex Scramble 41

Low Carb Chili 43

Grilled Shrimp And Chicken 45

Bacon Wrapped Mini Meatloaves 47

Low Carb Lettuce Wraps 49

Delicious Chili Cheese Dogs 52

Moroccan Style Chicken 56

Beef And Broccoli Stir Fry 58

Low Fat Mocha Frappie 60

Vanilla Oatmeal Shake 62

Grilled Chicken Salad 63

Salmon Patties 66

Chocolate-Hazelnut Protein Waffles 67

The Gluten-Free Coconut And Almond Bread 70

Avocado Egg Salad 72

Zucchini Frittata 74

Cream Cheese Clouds 76

Cream Cheese Peanut Butter Fat Bombs 77

Avocado Baked With Egg And Bacon 79

Mushroom And Ham Omelet 81

Cowboy Breakfast Skillet 83

Sausage And Egg Breakfast Bites 85

Fried Egg With Red Wine Vinegar 87

Salami Roll Ups 89

Mexican Veal Sausages 90

Crispy Caritas 92

Pizza Topping Casserole 95

Chocolate-Berry Protein Oatmeal 98

Stuffed Chicken Breast 99

Cherry Mango Smoothie 101

Orange Splash Apple-Avocado Shake 103

Low-Carb Almond Shortbread Cookies 104

Cinnamon And Cardamom Fat Bombs 106

Lemon Poppy Seed Protein Muffins............................. 108

Eggplant Mozzarella Casserole...................................... 111

Green Chile Frittata 114

Crisp Meringue Cookies 116

Double Chocolate Bundt Cake 119

Fried Egg With Ham And Broccoli 122

Rocket And Tomato Salad With Mozzarella................. 124

Coconut Oil-Fried Eggs And Vegetables 126

Mexican Veal Sausages 127

Carolina Style Barbeque Meatballs 129

Cheese Enchiladas... 132

Swedish Meatballs 136

Russian Stir-Fry.. 139

Chicken Breast Mushroom Sandwich........................... 140

Strawberry Greek Yogurt Whip 142

Winter Sunshine Smoothie 143

Beef Goulash

Ingredients:

- 1 sweet ball pepper, cubed
- 3 oz. onions chopped
- 1 tablespoon of chili salsa
- 3 tablespoons of cooking oil
- 2 1bs beef cubed, in 1 ½ inch cubes
- Salt and pepper
- Water
- 1 cup of red wine
- 1 1b of tomatoes, cubed

Directions:

1. Cubed beef should be fryed in a large pot or skillet in cooking oil

2. When the beef gets brown, chili salsa should be added and will be fryed for 1 minute
3. Onions and cubed vegetables should be added and frying will be continued for about 10 minutes
4. Wine and water can be added if needed
5. Get it covered and allow it to simmer for about 30 minutes
6. Add salt and pepper to taste

Upside down Breakfast Soufflé

Ingredients:

- ½ cup of thinly sliced mushroom
- 3 tablespoons of unsalted butter
- ½ cup of egg whites
- Cheese of your choice, ½
- Salt and pepper to taste
- ½ medium tomatoes, thinly sliced

Directions:
1. Oven should be preheated to 400 degrees
2. Salt and pepper should be added to giving egg whites and whip into soft peaks
3. In a cast iron skillet, the butter should be heated over high heat and get mushroom sauté till it becomes soft
4. Tomato slice should be placed over mushroom

5. Cheese should be quickly folded into egg whites mixture and will be poured on top of the mushroom/tomato mixture
6. Pan should then be placed in an oven and will be baked for about 8 minutes
7. Remove from oven and flip soufflé over onto serving plate

Low Carb Pancake Crepes

Ingredients:

- 1/2 teaspoon ground cinnamon
- 1 egg, beaten
- 1 and 1/2 teaspoons sugar free syrup
- 1/2 teaspoon butter
- 1 and 1/2 ounces cream cheese, softened

Directions:

1. Place the beaten egg in a medium sized bowl.
2. Add in about one tablespoon of cream cheese and mash using the back of a spoon until smooth and lump free.
3. Continue adding the cream cheese until it forms a smooth mixture.
4. Pour in the sugar free syrup and mix well. Add in the cinnamon and mix well.
5. Place the butter in a non-stick skillet and heat over a medium high flame.

6. Once the butter has melted, lower the heat to a medium low and add in a few tablespoons of the prepared cream cheese and egg mix.
7. Swirl the pan until the mixture coats the bottom of the skillet.
8. Let the batter cook untouched until it is set. It should take about 4 minutes.
9. Flip over using a spatula and cook on the other side until the crepe is lightly browned.
10. Serve immediately.
11. Enjoy!

Baby Spinach Omelet

Ingredients:

- 1/2 teaspoon onion powder
- Salt, to taste
- 1/4 teaspoon ground nutmeg
- Pepper, to taste
- 4 eggs
- 3 tablespoons grated Parmesan cheese
- 2 cups baby spinach leaves, torn into bite sized pieces

Directions:

1. Place the eggs in a medium bowl and beat well until lightly frothy.
2. Add in the baby spinach leaves and the grated Parmesan and mix well.
3. Add in the nutmeg, salt, onion powder and pepper.

4. Mix well to ensure that there are now lumps of spices.
5. Spray a medium skillet with some cooking spray and heat over a medium high flame until lightly smoking.
6. Pour in the egg mixture and swirl the pan around until it coats the bottom of the skillet.
7. Cook the mixture for about 3 minutes or until it is partially set.
8. Carefully flip over the omelet using a spatula and continue cooking the egg for another 3 to 4 minutes or until set.
9. Lower the heat to medium low and let the egg cook for another 2 minutes or until it reaches the desired level of doneness.
10. Serve immediately.
11. Enjoy!

Ground Beef With Sliced Bell Peppers

Ingredients:

- ½ cup Spinach, thinly sliced
- 1 bell pepper, thinly sliced
- Salt, to taste
- Pepper, to taste
- Cayenne, to taste
- 1 tablespoon Coconut Oil
- 1 Onion, finely chopped
- ½ lb. Ground Beef

Directions:

1. Pour the coconut oil into a pan and heat on a medium high flame until heated through.
2. Add in the onion and cook until the onion is translucent.

3. Once the onion is cooked, add in the ground beef and mix well until well browned.
4. Season with spices according to taste.
5. Top with the spinach and belle pepper and cook uncovered, constantly stirring until cooked through.
6. Serve hot.
7. Enjoy!

Garlic Lime Chicken Fajitas

Ingredients:

- 3 tbsp. lime juice
- 1tbsp orange juice
- 2 bundles stevia
- 2 tbsp. coconut oil
- ½ tsp. ocean salt
- 1.5 lbs. boneless skinless chicken bosom cut into slim strips
- 1 red pepper
- 1 green pepper
- 1 yellow onion
- 1 tsp. Dried out minced garlic
- 1 tsp. dried out mined onion
- 1 tsp. ground cumin
- 1 tsp. dried oregano

- 2 tbsp. new cilantro (or 1 tsp. dry cilantro)
- ½ tsp. coarse dark pepper

Directions:

1. Combine every one of the fixings with the exception of the peppers and onion in a huge bowl and blend until the chicken is completely coated.
2. Refrigerate something like 30 minutes so the chicken is well marinated.
3. Once the chicken has been marinated, heat a huge non-stick skillet on medium high hotness and sautéed food the chicken for a couple of moments until daintily brown.
4. Eliminate from container and set aside.
5. Add peppers and onion and cook for around 5 minutes or until tender.
6. Add the chicken to the pepper and onion blend for a couple of more minutes until completely cooked.

Protein Waffles

Ingredients:

- 2 scoops of Whey Protein Isolate (any flavor)
- 4 egg whites
- ½ cup Oats, mixed into flour
- 2 parcels of Stevia
- 1 tsp. Cinnamon
- 1 tsp. Coconut Oil

Directions:
1. Beat the egg whites
2. Add cinnamon, oat flour, stevia and cinnamon and blend well
3. Cook on a preheated waffle producer showered with Pam for 3 minutes
4. Meanwhile, blend all the fixing Ingredients:
5. Once the waffles are prepared, pour the fixing over them and enjoy!

The Amazing Low Carb Goulash (Hungarian Stew) Recipe

Ingredients:

- 2 lbs. (1") cubed veal
- 2 onions, white or yellow hacked finely (the better the better!)
- 2-3 garlic cloves minced
- 2tbsp Coconut Oil
- 2-3 Tbsp. (conform to taste) Hungarian sweet paprika
- 1 tsp. cove leaves
- 1 Qt. water or stock
- 1 head cauliflower
- ¼ tsp. dark pepper
- 1 tsp. salt
- 2 tsp. caraway seeds

Directions:

1. Add 1 tbsp. of oil or margarine to enormous pot and earthy colored meat on high hotness (only the outside of the meat should be cooked, this will assist with keeping the flavor and keep it sodden). Set aside
2. Add 1 tbsp. of oil to a skillet and fry onions on medium hotness until soft.
3. Add garlic until browned.
4. Bring the pot with meat back to the oven and add the singed onions and garlic to it and set on medium heat.
5. Add all flavors to water or stock.
6. Cook for around 1.5 to 2 hrs. (for hamburger or veal), and 20-25mins for chicken.
7. The more you cook the meat or veal the more delicate it will be.
8. The fluid will become thicker.

Vanilla-Pumpkin Protein Smoothie

Ingredients:

- Ice cubes 1 cup
- Pumpkin pie spice ¼ tsp
- Cinnamon ¼ tsp
- Vanilla whey protein powder ¼ cup
- Pumpkin Bits ⅓ cup
- Soy milk ¾ cup
- Vanilla Greek frozen yogurt ½ cup
- Frozen banana 1

Directions:

1. Place all of the Ingredients: into your blender and mix on high for around two to three minutes, or until it is smooth. Scrape the sides down as needed.
2. Add a little extra milk if your mixture is too thick. If it's too thin, add extra ice cubes.

Orangey Apple-Veggie Drink

Ingredients:

- Large lemon 1
- Large cucumber 1
- Medium apples 3
- Romaine lettuce – 150g
- Small Mandarin oranges 3
- Lime 1

Directions:

1. Wash all of the fruits and veggies very well. This is because you are going to be using the skins as well.
2. Run the fruits and veggies through your juicer. This will make 32 ounces of juice.
3. Mix well and serve. Sweeten with a calorie-free sweetener if desired.

Low-Carb Mashed Cauliflower

Ingredients:

- 2 cloves garlic, minced
- 1 teaspoon seasoned salt (such as LAWRY'S®), or to taste
- 1 head cauliflower, cut into florets
- ½ cup whipped cream cheese

Directions:

1. Bring a large pot of lightly salted water to a boil.
2. Cook cauliflower in boiling water until tender, about 6 minutes; drain.
3. Pat cauliflower dry with paper towel to remove as much moisture as possible.
4. Blend cauliflower, cream cheese, garlic, and seasoned salt in a food processor until mostly smooth.

Low-Carb Chicken and Mushroom Soup

Ingredients:

- 3 cups chicken stock
- 3 tablespoons chopped fresh tarragon, divided
- salt and freshly ground black pepper to taste
- 2 cups heavy whipping cream
- ½ cup butter
- 1 cooked chicken breast, cubed
- 1 small white onion, finely chopped
- 3 cloves garlic, finely chopped
- 1 ½ pounds fresh mushrooms, sliced

Directions:
1. Melt butter in a Dutch oven over medium-high heat. Add chicken; saute until lightly browned, about 3 minutes.

2. Add onion and garlic; saute until softened, about 5 minutes.
3. Stir in mushrooms; saute until tender, 5 to 10 minutes.
4. Pour in chicken stock and 2 tablespoons tarragon; reduce heat to low.
   Season with salt. Cover and simmer soup until flavors are combined, about 25 minutes.
5. Step 2
6. Stir cream into the soup; cook until heated through but not boiling.
7. Serve soup with pepper and the remaining tarragon on top.

White Bread

Ingredients:

- 2 cups water
- 1/2 cup oat bran
- 4 Tbsp psyllium husks
- 1 1/2 cup crucial wheat gluten
- 1 cup vanilla enhanced whey protein powder
- 3/4 cup rice protein powder
- 2 tsp salt
- 2 Tbsp oil
- 2 Tbsp Splenda
- 4 Tbsp yeast

Directions:
1. Pour every one of the fixings into a bread machine and cycle based on the maker's instructions.

2. Remove the portion and put away to cool.

Peach and Sour Cream Muffins

Ingredients:

- 1/2 cup sharp cream
- 1/4 cup softened butter
- 1 Tbsp cream
- 2 eggs
- 1 tsp orange peel
- 3/4 cup somewhat defrosted and diced frozen peaches
- 1/2 cup of soy flour
- 1/2 cup of vanilla protein powder
- 1/2 tsp baking powder
- 1/4 tsp salt
- 1/4 tsp baking soda
- 1 Tbsp Stevia-FOS blend

Directions:

1. Preheat broiler to 350o F (180 o C).
2. In a blending bowl, join the dry fixings in a little bowl.
3. In a different bowl, consolidate the margarine, cream, acrid cream, egg, and orange peel.
4. Add the peaches to the dry fixings then, at that point, consolidate the dry with the wet fixings. Blend until well distributed.
5. Line a biscuit tin with paper cups and spoon your player to fill the tin.
6. Heat for 20 to 25 minutes.

The Coconut Macadamia Bars

Ingredients:

- ¼ of a cup of a cup of coconut oil
- 5 tbsp. of shredded unsweetened coconut
- 15 drops of sweet leaf stevia.
- 2 cups or 60 grams of Macadamia nuts
- ½ a cup of almond butter

Directions:
1. Get a food processor or with the aid of your hand, only crush the macadamia nuts.
2. Get a mixing bowl, and inside combine the almond butter with the coconut oil, and shredded coconut.
3. Add the stevia drops as well as the crushed macadamia nuts.
4. Mix the batter very well before pouring it into a baking dish that has been lined with a parchment paper.

5. Bake for about 15 minutes, then cool and serve immediately.
6. Otherwise, you can store inside the refrigerator.

Low Carb, Paleo, Grain-Free Flax Waffles

Ingredients:

- 1 tsp. of lemon juice or apple cider vinegar
- ½ a tsp. of baking soda
- ½ a tsp. of vanilla extract
- ½ a tsp. of sea salt
- ½ cup of golden flax seed meal (ground)
- 2 medium to large pastured eggs
- 1 tsp. of coconut oil
- 2 tbsp. of milk (dairy free)
- You need a spray for your waffle maker; this could be olive oil.

Directions:

1. Heat your waffle maker up by plugging it, and then get a bowl where you can mix the Ingredients: until a smooth batter is created.

2. You may want to add an extra milk just to make it more seamless.
3. Once you get the green light from the waffle maker, you spray it with the olive oil with the aid of a master.
4. Add the batter and follow further instructions on the waffle maker. The battery should provide up to 5 waffles (Belgian style).
5. You can top up the waffles with some blueberries, and a dollop of coconut whip.
6. You may also top them up with some berry jam or maple syrup to create a delicious breakfast.

Broccoli Cheddar Soup

Ingredients:

- 1/2 cup heavy cream
- 1 1/2 cup vegetable broth
- 1 cup cheddar cheese
- 1 1/2 cup broccoli florets, steamed
- 4 oz cream cheese
- Dash salt

Directions:

1. Steam the broccoli until tender. Mix 1/2 cup of broccoli, all of cream cheese and all of cream in blender until smooth.
2. Pour mixture into a pot and add the rest of the Ingredients:, except the cheese.
3. Heat over medium heat until it comes to a simmer.

4. Once heated, add the cheddar cheese and mix until melted completely.

Onion Soup

Ingredients:

- 1 celery stalk chopped
- 2 cups chicken broth
- 4 tbsp of butter
- Thyme and pepper to taste
- 1/2 onion chopped
- 4 cups of mushrooms, chopped
- 1 clove garlic chopped

Directions:
1. Put butter in pot on medium heat.
2. When melted add onion, garlic, and celery.
3. Cooked until softened, add mushrooms, thyme and pepper.

4. Let cook for a few minutes then add chicken broth.
5. Add water 2 cups of water. Let mixture heat on medium heat for about 15 minutes.
6. With blender, blend until desired consistency. Add in cream and blend.

Coconut White Chocolate Fudge

Ingredients:

- 1/2 cup of Vanilla Protein Powder
- 1/2 cup of Coconut Oil
- 1 cup of Coconut Butter
- 15-ounce container of Coconut Milk 1 teaspoon of Vanilla Extract Pinch of Salt
- 4 ounces of Cacao Butter
- 1 teaspoon of Coconut Liquid Stevia
- Optional: Unsweetened Coconut Flake

Directions:

1. Melt your cacao margarine in your pan over a low heat.
2. Stir in your coconut milk, coconut oil, and coconut butter.

3. Continue to mix until totally smooth, no lumps.
4. Turn off your hotness and speed in protein powder, vanilla concentrate, stevia, and salt.
5. Pour your combination into a material fixed 8x8 pan.
6. Sprinkle with coconut drops if desired.
7. Refrigerate for 4 hours or overnight.
8. Shouldn't be kept refrigerated for storage.

Coffee Cake Cinnamon Collagen Fat Bombs

Ingredients:

- 1 tablespoon of Instant Coffee
- 1 bundle of Vanilla Collagen
- 1 teaspoon of Cinnamon
- 1/4 cup of Almond Butter
- 1/2 cup of Coconut Oil

Directions:

1. In your little measured pot heat coconut oil and almond spread on low until melted.
2. Microwave your coconut oil for around 30 seconds until melted.
3. Stir together all of your Ingredients:.
3. Pour into a 8x8 skillet, smaller than usual biscuit tins, or silicone/plastic sweets molds. Freeze until firm.

Scrambled eggs with bacon and chard

Ingredients:

- 20g cherry tomatoes
- 3 eggs size m
- 1 tbsp cream
- 50g bacon
- 20g swiss chard
- Some walnut oil
- Sea salt and pepper

Directions:

1. Wash the chard and cherry tomatoes and dry them well. Halve the cherry tomatoes.
2. Then whisk the three eggs together with the cream in a bowl. Season with sea salt and pepper to taste.
3. Heat the oil in a pan, fry the bacon until crispy and then place on a kitchen towel.

4. Pour the egg-cream mixture into the pan you have just used and fry, turning occasionally, until the eggs are done.
5. Arrange the scrambled eggs together with the halved tomatoes, the Swiss chard and the bacon on a plate. Pour a few dashes of oil over the cherry tomatoes and chard, then season with sea salt and pepper to taste.

Avocado Chicken Omelet

Ingredients:

- 70g paprika (red)
- 15g parsley
- 3 eggs size m
- 1 tbsp cream
- 130g avocado
- 100g chicken breast
- 70g paprika (green)
- Some olive oil
- Sea salt and pepper

Directions:
1. First cut the chicken breast into large pieces and then put it in a pan with a little olive oil and fry it until crispy.
2. Season to taste with salt and pepper.

3. Then wash the two peppers, cut in half and cut into cubes.
4. Wash the avocado, cut in half and remove half of the skin. Then cut into strips approx. 1 cm thick.
5. Then wash the parsley, shake it dry and chop it finely. Cut the chicken breast fillet into strips.
6. Whisk the eggs together with the cream in a bowl and season with sea salt and pepper.
7. Heat the oil in a pan and add the egg mixture. As soon as the mixture has hardened, turn it carefully.
8. Place the finished omelet on a plate and place the chicken breast strips together with the avocado strips in the middle.
9. Close the omelet and add the diced paprika. Drizzle with a little olive oil.
10. Garnish with salt, pepper and the parsley.

Cheese Chive Waffles

Ingredients:

- 2 eggs
- 1 teaspoon onion powder
- 1 teaspoon garlic powder
- ½ teaspoon pepper
- 1 tablespoon chives
- 1 cup raw cauliflower (cut into small pieces)
- 1 cup mozzarella cheese (shredded)
- 1/3 cup Parmesan cheese (shredded)
- Optional: fresh parsley
- Optional: Sun-dried tomatoes

Directions:
1. Mix Ingredients: into a batter.
2. Heat the waffle maker until it's ready.
3. Add batter in batches of ¼ cups each.

4. Set the timer at 4-6 minutes.
5. Take a peek after the fourth minute. If the maker sticks, cook for a few more minutes.
6. Once cooked, put in on a plate and allow it to cool.
7. Put any remaining batter in the refrigerator.

Tex Mex Scramble

Ingredients:

- ½ cup frozen spinach (thawed and drained)
- 5 slices Jalapeno pepper (chopped)
- 1 slice pepper jack or cheddar cheese
- 2 tablespoons Pace Salsa
- 5 Eggs
- 2 tablespoons water
- 1/8 cup green pepper (chopped)
- 1/8 cup red onion (chopped)
- 2 cherry tomatoes (diced)

Directions:

1. Preheat the skillet at medium heat. Put in oil.
2. Mix eggs with water, onion, pepper, spinach, tomatoes, and jalapenos.

3. Pour them into the skillet. Cook until the eggs reach your preferred consistency.
4. Just a little before the eggs are ready, turn the heat off and add the cheese.
5. Cover and let the mixture sit for around 5 minutes.
6. Put salsa on top before serving.

Low Carb Chili

Ingredients:

- 2 bay leaves
- 2 teaspoons of salt
- 4 cups of canned tomatoes, drained
- 2 1bs lean beef, chopped
- 3 tablespoons of olive oil
- 2 cans of Eden Black soybeans, drained
- 2 to 3 tablespoons of chili powder
- ¼ teaspoon of crushed cumin
- 1 teaspoon of oregano
- 2 cloves of minced garlic

Directions:

1. All Ingredients: should be placed in a stock pot
2. Bring to a boil, get heat reduced and simmer for 1 to 2 hours

3. The longer it simmers, the more the flavor sets in
4. For cab reduction, beef broth should be substituted for tomatoes

Grilled Shrimp and Chicken

Ingredients:

- ½ pint of heavy cream
- 2 tablespoons of butter
- 1 tablespoon of garlic powder
- 1/8 teaspoon of onion powder
- 1/8 teaspoon of white pepper
- 1/8 to ¼ teaspoon of cayenne pepper
- ½ teaspoon of poultry seasoning
- Grated Romano cheese for garnish
- 8 ounces shrimp
- 4 skinless, boneless chicken breasts
- ½ cup of white wine
- 1 tablespoon of olive oil
- ½ cup of chicken broth

Directions:
1. All poultry seasoning should be combined together in a small bowl and will be divided into ½
2. Butter should be melted in the skillet over low heat add cream broth, and ½ spice mixture
3. Stirring should be vigorous and be allowed to sauce well and be set aside
4. Grill should be preheated to high heat
5. Cooking oil should be heating over high heat in a large skillet
6. Chicken breast and wine should be added and sauté with the remaining ½ of spice mixture till the chicken gets cooked through
7. Put down from heat and set aside
8. Lightly oil grill grates, shrimp should be placed on hot grill and will be cooked for about 3 to 4 minutes

9. Each chicken breast will be served topped with grilled shrimp and will be covered with cream sauce

Bacon Wrapped Mini Meatloaves

Ingredients:

- 1 garlic clove, minced
- Fresh parsley, chopped
- Freshly ground black pepper, to taste
- Salt, to taste
- 1/2 lb. ground beef
- 4 additional strips of bacon
- 1/4 lb. bacon, cut in small chunks
- 2 tablespoons coconut milk
- 3 tablespoons fresh chives, minced

Directions:

1. Crank up your oven to 400 degrees F and allow the oven to preheat.
2. Combine the ground beef, garlic, coconut milk, bacon chunks and chives together in a large mixing bowl using a wooden spoon or an electric mixer. Keep mixing until the Ingredients: hold together.
3. Season with salt and pepper to taste. (Use a low amount of salt as the bacon is already salted)
4. In a medium sized muffin tin, place the bacon on the sides of the mold.
5. Fill the same four molds with the prepared beef mixture.
6. Pop the muffin tray into the preheated oven and bake for about 30 to 35 minutes.
7. Once cooked through, remove the muffin tin from the oven and cool for about 10 minutes or until the muffins are cool enough to handle.

8. De-mold the mini meatloaves and serve immediately topped with some fresh parsley.
9. Enjoy!

Low Carb Lettuce Wraps

Ingredients:

- Handful of cilantro, chopped
- 2 tablespoons low sodium soy sauce
- Juice of ½ lemon
- ½ teaspoon chili garlic sauce
- Iceberg lettuce
- ½ teaspoon sesame oil
- ½ avocado, sliced
- 1 ½ tablespoons fat of your choice, preferably olive oil or coconut oil
- 2 oz. shiitake mushrooms, chopped

- 1/2 lb. boneless and skinless chicken breasts, chopped into tiny cubes
- 1/4 onion diced
- 1 green onion, finely chopped
- 2 cloves garlic, minced

Directions:

1. Place about 1 tablespoon of the fat of your choice in a small sauté pan and heat on a medium low flame until lightly smoking.
2. Add the chicken to the pan and toss well until cooked through.
3. While the chicken is sizzling in the pan, place the lemon juice, soy sauce, green onion, chili garlic sauce, sesame oil and cilantro together in a mixing bowl.
4. Once the chicken is done, add it to the bowl and mix well.

5. While the chicken cooks, add the chili sauce, lemon juice, sesame oil, soy sauce, green onions and cilantro into a serving bowl.
6. Once the chicken is done, add it to the bowl.
7. Add the remaining fat to the sauté pan and heat. Once smoking, add in the onion, mushrooms and garlic to it. Sauté for about 10 minutes or until cooked through.
8. Empty the contents of the sauté pan into the mixing bowl and toss well to coat.
9. Carefully cut away the stem of the lettuce. Remove individual lettuce leaves and wash well.
10. Make small "cups" out of the lettuce and spoon some of the prepared chicken filling into the lettuce cup.
11. Serve immediately topped with a slice of avocado.
12. Enjoy!

Delicious Chili Cheese Dogs

Ingredients:

- ½ 15 oz. can fire roasted tomatoes, drained out of the liquid, chopped finely
- ¼ red onion, diced
- ½ tablespoon chili powder
- 1 clove of garlic, minced
- ¼ teaspoon cocoa powder (optional)
- 1 ½ sweet potatoes, cut into halves length wise
- 3 low fat, low sodium hot dogs
- 2 tablespoons Olive oil + oil for dousing sweet potatoes
- ½ lb. ground beef
- 1 Chipotle pepper soaked in adobe sauce, chopped

- Pepper, to taste
- Salt, to taste
- 1 ½ oz. sharp cheddar cheese, grated

Directions:

1. Crank up your oven to 450 degrees F and allow the oven to preheat.
2. Douse your sweet potato halves with a healthy amount of olive oil.
3. Place the oil-covered sweet potatoes on a baking sheet with their skin side up.
4. Pop the baking sheet into the preheated oven and bake for about 30 minutes or until the skin is crispy and the insides soften.
5. While the sweet potatoes bake, add 2 tablespoons olive oil into a sauté pan. Hat on a medium low flame until lightly smoking.
6. Add in the onions and garlic and sauté for about 10 minutes or until softened.

7. Add in the tomatoes, cocoa powder, chipotle peppers, chili powder, salt and pepper. Mix well to combine.
8. Crumble the ground beef into the pan, ensuring there are no large chunks of ground beef in the pan.
9. Continue cooking the chili until all the components of the chili are cooked thoroughly.
10. Once the sweet potatoes are cooked, remove them from the baking sheet.
11. Place the hot dogs on the baking sheet and pop them into the still hot oven for about 7 minutes.
12. Spoon out the mushy center of the sweet potatoes and save the sweet potato mush for future use.
13. To assemble your Chili Cheese Dogs place the crisp sweet potato skins on a serving plate.

14. Place the hot dog on the crispy skin, spoon some prepared chili onto it and sprinkle some grated cheese over the chili.
15. Serve immediately.
16. Enjoy!

Moroccan Style Chicken

Ingredients:

- 1 tbsp. cumin powder
- 2 cloves of minced garlic
- 3 tbsp. of olive oil (optional)
- ½ cup red wine vinegar
- 1-2 medium onions cut into long meager strips
- ½ tsp. cinnamon powder
- 1 tbsp. stew powder
- 1 tsp. paprika
- 8 (125g every) chicken skinless boneless chicken breasts

Directions:

1. Preheat stove 350ºF.

2. Combine every one of the flavors along with oil and vinegar and combine or mix as one to make marinade.
3. Chop onions longwise into rings and set aside.
4. Place chicken bosoms in a profound baking container (ideally one that accompanies a lid)
5. Pour marinade over chicken (it's far superior assuming you let the chicken marinade in the cooler for a couple of hours, however works regardless) and add the onions.
6. Make sure that the chicken is uniformly covered with marinade onions.
7. Bake for 1 hour or until chicken is done (check and turn pieces following 25 minutes and afterward check each 10 min).

Beef and Broccoli Stir Fry

Ingredients:

- 10 oz. sirloin steak cut into strips
- 6 tbsp. low sodium chicken or meat broth
- 2 tbsp. decreased sodium soy sauce
- 1 tsp. corn starch
- 2 bundle Stevia
- 2 tsp. coconut oil
- 6 cups broccoli cut into florets
- 4 meagerly cut carrot
- 2 onions, cut into flimsy wedges

Directions:

1. Heat coconut oil in an enormous skillet and add the hacked vegetables.

2. Sauté until veggies are fresh, delicate and onions are caramelized. Set aside.
3. Stir in the meat strips, cook until wanted tenderness.
4. In a different bowl, join stock, soy sauce, cornstarch, and stevia mixing to disintegrate the cornstarch completely.
5. Add to the hamburger and veggie combination and cook blending continually until sauce thickens.

Low Fat Mocha Frappie

Ingredients:

- Liquid sweetener 3 drops
- 0% Fat Greek yogurt ½ cup
- Unsweetened almond milk ¼ cup
- Brewed coffee – ½ cup
- Low-sugar chocolate syrup (optional)
- Low-fat whipped cream (optional)
- Ice 1 cup
- Cocoa powder 1 tbs

Directions:

1. Add the ice, cocoa, sweetener, yogurt, milk, and coffee to your blender and pulse it a few times to mix everything together extremely well.

2. Pour your mix into a tall glass and top it with some whipped cream and chocolate syrup if desired. Enjoy.

Vanilla Oatmeal Shake

Ingredients:

- Low-fat nut milk 1 cup
- Vanilla whey protein powder 1 scoop
- Vanilla extract ¼ tsp
- Oatmeal 1 tbs
- Ground cinnamon ½ tsp

Directions:

1. Add the extract, oatmeal, cinnamon, milk, and protein powder to a blender.
2. Mix everything together. If you want your shake to be thicker, you can add some ice.
3. Pour the shake into a glass. If you want, you can serve it with a dusting of cinnamon, berries as garnish, or a squirt of low-fat whip cream.

Grilled Chicken Salad

Ingredients:

- 3/4 cup slashed red cabbage
- 1/6 cup canned pineapple lumps in juice, diced into little pieces 1/4 cup salsa
- 3 Tbsp Teriyaki sauce
- Lime and Mustard Dressing
- 3/4 lb boneless, skinless chicken breast
- 2 cups ice sheet lettuce, chopped
- 2 cups cleaved leaf lettuce

Teriyaki sauce:

- 1 clove garlic, crushed
- 1 Tbsp Splenda
- 1/2 Tbsp ground new ginger root
- 1/4 cup soy sauce
- 1/8 cup dry sherry

Lime and Mustard Dressing:

- 3/4 Tbsp maple syrup
- 3/4 Tbsp canola oil
- 3/4 Tbsp juice vinegar
- 3/4 Tbsp lime juice
- 1/8 cup Dijon mustard
- 1/8 cup Splenda

Directions:

Teriyaki sauce:

1. Mix every one of the fixings together in a bowl.
2. Honey Lime and Mustard Dressing:
3. In a bowl, whisk every one of the fixings together.

Barbecued chicken salad:

1. Marinate the chicken in the Teriyaki sauce inside the fridge for something like 2 hours and ideally overnight.

2. In a plate of mixed greens bowl, join the ice shelf and leaf lettuces, red cabbage, and pineapple bits.
3. Prepare your chicken for barbecuing by depleting the marinade into a bowl and barbecuing the chicken, seasoning it with the marinade.
4. Cook on the two sides for 3 to 5 minutes or until all around good done. Cut cooked chicken into pieces.
5. Toss the plate of mixed greens with the Lime and Mustard Dressing.
6. Circulate salad between two plates and top with cut barbecued chicken.
7. Spoon salsa on top of the chicken and serve.

Salmon Patties

Ingredients:

- 8 oz salmon
- 1/8 cup oat bran
- 1/2 beaten egg
- 1 scallion, finely sliced
- 1 1/2 Tbsp margarine

Directions:

1. Drain the salmon and squash it in a blending bowl.
2. Add the egg, oat wheat, and scallions. Blend well and structure 6 to 8 patties.
3. Place a weighty skillet over medium hotness and soften the margarine.
4. Saute the salmon patties, making a point to turn once and cautiously.
5. Cook for 7 minutes per side or until golden.

Chocolate-Hazelnut Protein Waffles

Ingredients:

- 4 eggs
- 1/3 of a cup of Greek yoghurt (Full fat)
- 2 2/3 tbsp. Of hazelnut oil
- ½ tsp. Of hazelnut extract
- ¼ tbsp. Of extract of stevia.
- 1 ¼ cups of Hazelnut meal
- ½ a cup of chocolate protein powder
- 2 tbsp. Of cocoa powder
- 2 tbsp. Of coconut flour
- 3 tbsp. Of swerve natural sweetener (a granulated erythritol)

Directions:

1. Preheat the waffle iron to meat, and then pre-heat the oven to about 200 degrees F.

2. place a wire rack on top of the baking sheet.
3. Get a large bowl, and inside, whisk together the protein powder, alongside the hazelnut meal, sweetener, coconut flour and the cocoa powder.
4. Get another small to medium bowl and inside, whisk the egg alongside the yogurt, hazelnut oil, stevia and hazelnut extract and mix perfectly well until they are appropriately combined.
5. If necessary, you can grease the waffle iron and then pour a quarter of the batter into each section of the waffle iron, close the waffle iron, and then cook the waffles until they become light brown and crispy in texture.
6. Gently transfer the cooked waffles onto the baking sheet in the oven to keep them warm.
7. Cook the remaining batter inside the waffle iron and then transfer them to the oven.

8. Top up the waffles with butter, berries, whipped cream, sugar-free syrup, and serve.

The Gluten-Free Coconut and Almond Bread

Ingredients:

- 4-5 large eggs
- ¼ of a cup of coconut oil
- 1 tsp. of a natural sweetener such as stevia
- 1 tbsp. of apple cider vinegar
- 1 3/4 tbsp. of almond flour
- 1 ½ tbsp. of coconut flour
- ¼ of a cup of ground flaxseed
- ¼ tbsp. of salt
- 1 tsp. of baking soda

Directions:

1. Pre-heat the oven to about 350 degrees F, and then grease the loaf of the pan.

2. Mix the almond, and coconut flour, alongside the flaxseed, salt, and baking soda, inside a food processor.
3. Pulse the Ingredients: together, before you add the eggs, vinegar, and oil.
4. Pour the mix or batter into the loaf pan, and bake for about 30 minutes at the 350 degrees F in the oven.
5. Let the bread cool for few minutes before serving.

Avocado Egg Salad

Ingredients:

- 1 teaspoon prepared yellow mustard
- 1/4 teaspoon paprika
- salt and ground black pepper to taste
- 8 eggs
- 1/2 avocado, peeled and pitted
- 1/4 cup chopped green onion (optional)

Directions:

1. Place eggs in a saucepan and cover with water.
2. Bring to a boil, remove from heat, and let eggs stand in hot water for 15 minutes.
3. Remove eggs from hot water, cool under cold running water, and peel.
4. Chop eggs and transfer to a salad bowl.
5. Mash avocado in a separate bowl using a fork.

6. Mix mashed avocado, yellow mustard, and paprika into eggs until thoroughly combined.
7. Season with salt and black pepper.

Zucchini Frittata

Ingredients:

- 2 green onions, thinly sliced, or to taste
- 2 cloves garlic, minced
- 1 teaspoon onion powder
- 1 teaspoon dried basil
- 1 teaspoon sea salt
- 3/4 teaspoon freshly ground black pepper
- 2 tablespoons coconut oil, melted
- 1 cup shredded zucchini
- 1 small yellow onion, or to taste, grated
- 6 large eggs
- 1/2 cup almond flour

Directions:

1. Preheat oven to 350 degrees F (175 degrees C). Grease a baking dish with coconut oil.

2. Drain zucchini and onion in a colander until no longer wet, about 10 minutes.
3. Beat eggs, almond flour, green onions, garlic, onion powder, basil, sea salt, and black pepper together in a large mixing bowl until smooth; stir zucchini and onion into the egg.
4. Pour the egg mixture into the prepared baking dish.
5. Bake in preheated oven until set in the center, 35 to 40 minutes.

Cream Cheese Clouds

Ingredients:

- 1/2 cup of Softened Unsalted Butter
- 3/4 cup of Granular Splenda
- 8 ounces of Softened Cream Cheese
- 1/2 teaspoon of Vanilla

Directions:

1. Beat everything with your electric blender until fluffy.
2. Drop scaled down spoonfuls onto your wax paper-lined baking sheet.
3. Freeze until firm, no less than 60 minutes.
4. Store in your cooler and eat frozen.

Cream Cheese Peanut Butter Fat Bombs

Ingredients:

- 1 tablespoon of Lemon Juice
- 3/4 cup of Almond Flour
- 1/4 cup of Swerve Icing
- 3/4 cup of Softened Peanut Butter
- 4 ounces of Softened Cream Cheese
- 2 tablespoons of Softened Butter

Directions:

1. Line 12 small biscuit tins with your paper liners and set aside.
2. You can likewise utilize your ice solid shape tray.
3. In your medium-sized bowl, join your relaxed cream cheddar, margarine, and peanut butter until totally smooth.

4. Add your almond flour, lemon juice, and sugar and rush until joined.
5. Equally convey into the pre-arranged biscuit tins.
6. Place in your cooler for somewhere around 60 minutes.
7. Once frozen, move the fat bombs to a Ziploc sack for better putting away.
8. Save them in the cooler for up to 3 months.

Avocado baked with egg and bacon

Ingredients:

- 25g gouda (grated)
- 2 eggs size m
- 250g avocado
- 100g bacon
- Some olive oil
- Sea salt and pepper

Directions:
1. Wash the avocado, cut in half and then remove the stone.
2. One egg comes into the recess of the core.
3. Depending on the size of the avocado, it has to be enlarged a little.
4. Excess pulp can be served with the cherry tomatoes at the end.

5. Place the two avocado halves on a baking sheet lined with baking paper. Preheat the oven to 180 ° C.
6. Cut the bacon into small cubes and fry in a heated pan. Then distribute evenly over the eggs. Sprinkle with grated cheese.
7. Season the two avocado halves with pepper and sea salt and then bake on the middle rack for about 15 minutes.
8. Take the avocado halves out of the oven and drizzle with a little walnut oil, olive oil or another oil as you like.

Mushroom and ham omelet

Ingredients:

- 10ml cream
- 10ml mineral water
- 4 eggs size m
- Some olive oil
- 100g cooked ham
- 70g mushrooms
- 15g parsley
- Sea salt and pepper

Directions:
1. Wash the parsley, shake dry and chop finely.
2. Then wash the mushrooms thoroughly and cut into thin slices.
3. Cut the cooked ham into cubes.
4. Then whisk the four eggs together with the cream and mineral water in a bowl.

5. Stir the parsley into the eggs, season with pepper and sea salt.
6. Heat the oil in the pan and fry the mushrooms.
7. Then take the mushrooms out of the pan and place on a kitchen towel.
8. Immediately afterwards add the egg mixture to the pan and cook over medium heat until the underside of the omelet is thick.
9. Carefully turn the omelet and finish cooking.
10. Finally, place the omelet on a plate, place the mushrooms and diced ham on top and close the omelet.

Cowboy Breakfast Skillet

Ingredients:

- 5 eggs
- 1 avocado (diced)
- A handful of cilantro
- Hot sauce
- 1 breakfast sausage (large)
- 2 sweet potatoes (diced, medium sized)
- Salt and pepper
- Optional: raw cheese

Directions:
1. Preheat the oven to 400 degrees F.
2. Over medium heat, crumble and fry the sausage. Be sure to use an oven-safe skillet.
3. Once the sausage turns brown, pick it up with a slotted spoon. Set it aside, making a point to

reserve the sausage grease in the skillet as much as possible.
4. Cook the sweet potatoes in the sausage grease until crispy.
5. Put the sausage back in the skillet.
6. Form wells in the skillet – one per egg. Put the eggs in these wells.
7. Put the skillet in the oven. Bake it just enough for the eggs to set.
8. Turn the oven to broil. Cook until the egg yolks are according to your preference.
9. Remove the skillet from the oven. Top with cilantro, avocado, and hot sauce.

Sausage and Egg Breakfast Bites

Ingredients:

- 1-2 cups, crumbled uncooked sausage
- 8-10 eggs
- 1 small bunch parsley
- 1 small bunch of Dark Greens – can be spinach, kale, beet greens, Swiss chard

Directions:

1. Preheat the oven to 375 degrees F.
2. Slice the greens so that they turn to thin strips. If you use kale, cut off the stem.
3. Sauté the greens in butter. Use medium heat.
4. Add the sausage after several minutes.
5. Sauté until sausage is cooked. Then, turn off the heat.
6. Whisk eggs. Add in the greens, parsley, and sausage. Stir them together.
7. Pour the mixture into a greased pan.

8. Bake for 20-25 minutes. Let it cool. Cut off into bite size squares before serving.

Fried Egg with Red Wine Vinegar

Ingredients:

- 1/8 teaspoon of pepper
- ½ teaspoon of salt
- 4 eggs
- 1 tablespoon of butter
- ½ teaspoon of parsley
- 2 teaspoons of red wine vinegar
- 1/8 teaspoon of marjoram

Directions:

1. Eggs should be broken into skillet over ½ tablespoon melted butter
2. Spices should then be added and will be cooked till whites becomes solid
3. Eggs should be placed onto serving plates
4. The remaining ½ teaspoon of butter will be melted and heated for about 2 minutes

5. Stirring in red wine vinegar will be done and the mixture will be allowed to cook for another 1 minute
6. Pour over eggs and then garnish with parsley

Salami Roll Ups

Ingredients:

- 1 tablespoon of cream cheese
- 5 large slices of hard salami
- 2 celery stalks

Directions:

1. Cream cheese should be soften in microwave and will be spread over salami, roll up
2. Celery will be enjoyed on the side

Mexican Veal Sausages

Ingredients:

- ½ teaspoon of ground cumin
- 2 tablespoons of green or red salsa
- 2 tablespoons of fresh cilantro, chopped
- 2 green onions, finely chopped, 1/3 cup
- 1 ½ pounds ground veal
- 1 lime, cut into slices for garnish
- ¼ cup of sour cream for garnish
- ¼ cup of green or red salsa for garnish
- 2 tablespoons of olive oil
- ¼ teaspoon freshly ground pepper
- ½ teaspoon of salt

Directions:

1. Onion, veal and all spices should be combined in a large mixing bowl and blended together

2. Mixture should then be shaped into 4 sausage links
3. Oil should be heated in a non-stick skillet on high heat and brown sausage to about 8 to 10 minutes, turning should be frequently done

Crispy Caritas

Ingredients:

- ½ teaspoon chili powder
- 1 bay leaf
- ½ cinnamon stick
- 2 garlic cloves, thinly sliced
- Water, for braising
- ½ onion, chopped or thinly sliced
- 2 pounds pork shoulder, cut into 5 pieces
- ½ teaspoon cumin
- ¾ teaspoon salt

Directions:

1. Crank up your oven to 350 ºF and allow the oven to preheat.

2. Combine the cumin, salt and chili powder together to make a spice rub. Rub it well onto the pork shoulder pieces.
3. In a large heavy bottomed pot, place the spice rubbed meat pieces along with the cinnamon stick, garlic, bay leaf and the onion. Try to make sure that your meat is in a single layer.
4. Pour some water over the meat, until the water level is almost, but not completely, covering the meat.
5. Place the pot into the oven uncovered and allow to braise for about 3 ½ to 4 hours. You will know your meat is cooked when it becomes extremely tender, browns and most of the braising liquid is gone.
6. Once the meat is cooked, carefully remove the pot from the oven. Using tongs remove the meat pieces onto a large cutting board and let it cool a bit, before slicing it into thin slices or shredding it using your hands.

7. Remove the bay leaf and cinnamon stick from the pot and add the thinly sliced or shredded meat into the pot. Return the pot into the oven.
8. Let the meat roast in the oven, stirring it with a wooden spoon occasionally, until the meat is crispy and becomes really dark. (If you wish to speed up the process, spread the meat and the liquid from the pot into a baking sheet and spread it into a single even layer. The meat will become crisp faster.)
9. Serve the crisp meat with low carb bread.
10. Enjoy!

Pizza Topping Casserole

Ingredients:

- ¼ teaspoon Italian seasoning
- ¼ cup green pepper, chopped
- 2 ounces pepperoni, chopped
- 4 ounces whole milk mozzarella cheese, cubed
- Crushed red pepper, optional
- 2 tablespoons olive oil
- ½ pound bulk Italian sausage, chopped into bite sized pieces
- 2 eggs
- 4 ounces fresh mushrooms, sliced
- ¼ cup heavy cream
- ¼ teaspoon garlic powder
- 2 tablespoons low sodium pizza sauce

- ¼ cup red onion, cut into thin slices

Directions:

1. Heat the olive oil in a sauté pan and heat over a medium high flame until lightly smoking. Add in the sausage and mushrooms and cook until the meat is well browned and the mushrooms are cooked through.
2. Place the eggs, pizza sauce, garlic powder, Italian seasoning, crushed red pepper and cream in a medium bowl. Whisk well to combine.
3. Grease a 7 x 12 inch shallow baking dish with some oil. Place the meats, peppers, mushrooms and mozzarella cubes in it. Pour the prepared egg mixture over it and mix well to combine.
4. Top with the sliced red onion.
5. Sprinkle a little more garlic powder, crushed red pepper flakes and Italian seasoning over the red onion.

6. Pop the baking dish into an oven and bake at 350 degrees F for 45 to 60 minutes or until the top is well browned and a skewer inserted in the center comes out almost clean.
7. Remove the pan from the oven and let it stand for about 5 minutes before cutting into bite sized pieces.
8. Serve hot.
9. Enjoy!

Chocolate-Berry Protein Oatmeal

Ingredients:

- 2 parcels of stevia
- 1 tbsp. of flax oil
- ½ cup of frozen mixed berries
- ¼ cup of water
- ½ cup dry oats
- 4 egg whites
- ½ scoop of whey protein isolate powder
- 1 tsp. of pure cocoa powder

Directions:

1. In a major bowl, blend every one of the fixings (aside from the frozen Berries).
2. Microwave on high setting for 1-2 minutes, until the oats is of a little runny consistency.

3. Once cooked, add the frozen berries, mix and appreciate.

Stuffed Chicken Breast

Ingredients:

- 3 cloves of minced garlic
- 1 huge onion
- 1 c Greek yogurt
- Salt and pepper (to taste)
- 4 4oz chicken breasts
- 2 c diced mushrooms
- 2 c new spinach
- 2 enormous diced tomatoes

Directions:
1. Spray Pam on a medium hotness skillet.
2. Add mushrooms, tomatoes, garlic, onions, Greek yogurt and spices.

3. Sautee the vegetables until delicate and the onions are translucent.
4. Cut the chicken bosoms evenly to shape a pocket in every single one of them.
5. Stuff every chicken bosom with new spinach and the sautéed vegetables.
6. Put in the broiler and prepare for 30-40 minutes on 400.
7. This formula works out positively on a bed of earthy colored rice.
8. In the event that a portion of the sautéed vegetables are left over you can place them on top of the rice, or simply eat them as an enhancement assuming you are cutting carbs.

Cherry Mango Smoothie

Ingredients:

- Water ½ cup
- Frozen sweeten cherries 1 cup
- Water ¾ cup
- Frozen mango 1 cup

Directions:

1. Allow the mangoes and cherries to sit in separate bowls until they are thawed, which should take around ten minutes.
2. Add the cherries to a blender with half a cup of water and blend until smooth.
3. Add in a little more water if it seems too thick. Pour the mixture into a glass.
4. Rinse out the blender and add in the mango and remaining water.
5. Blend until smooth, adding more water if you need to.

6. Pour this over the cherries and mix well.

Orange Splash Apple-Avocado Shake

Ingredients:

- Spinach leaves small handful
- Dessert pear 1
- Apple 1
- Orange juice ⅔ cup
- Chopped and peeled avocado ¼
- Low-fat coconut milk 5 tbs

Directions:
1. Core the pear and apple and dice them into small chunks.
2. Add them to the blender along with the orange juice, avocado, coconut milk, and spinach.
3. Pulse the mixture until everything is evenly mixed and smooth.
4. Pour into a glass and enjoy.

Low-Carb Almond Shortbread Cookies

Ingredients:

- 2 tablespoons butter, softened
- 1 egg white
- ¼ teaspoon vanilla extract
- ¾ cup almond flour
- 3 tablespoons granular no-calorie sucralose sweetener (such as Splenda®)
- 1 dash salt

Directions:

1. Mix almond flour, sweetener, and salt together in a small bowl with a fork.
2. Add butter, egg white, and vanilla extract; continue mixing with a fork.
3. Place in the freezer to help it harden for 15 minutes.

4. Meanwhile, preheat the oven to 325 degrees F (165 degrees C).
5. Line a baking sheet with parchment paper or use a silicone baking mat.
6. Remove batter from freezer. Measure out 1 teaspoon at a time; roll into balls and place on the prepared baking sheet.
7. Place plastic wrap on the bottom of a glass and roll dough balls flat.
8. Bake in the preheated oven until light, golden brown, 15 to 20 minutes.

Cinnamon and Cardamom Fat Bombs

Ingredients:

- ¼ of a tsp. of vanilla extract
- 1 tbsp. of ground cinnamon
- 3 oz. butter
- 5 tbsp. of unsweetened coconut (shredded)
- ½ tsp. of green ground Cardamom

Directions:

1. If the butter is not already stored at room temperature, make sure you bring it to the ideal temperature by removing it from the refrigerator.
2. Get a pan, and inside, simply roast the shredded coconut until it becomes brownish a little.
3. Roasting will help create an excellent flavor; however, you can skip this step and just allow the coconut to cool.

4. Mix the butter with the half of the shredded coconut alongside the spices, inside the bowl, and then form the mix into Walnut-size balls with the aid of a tsp., and roll the remaining shredded coconut inside.
5. Store the mix in the refrigerator or serve immediately.

Lemon Poppy Seed Protein Muffins

Ingredients:

- 1 tbsp. of lemon zest
- 1 tbsp. of coconut oil or melted unsalted butter
- 1 large egg stored at room temperature
- 1 tsp. of vanilla extract
- ¼ of a cup of pure and non-fat Greek yoghurt
- ¼ of cup of agave
- 2 tbsp. of freshly squeezed juice of lemon
- ½ a cup of unsweetened vanilla almond milk
- ½ a cup plus 2 tbsp. of coconut flour
- 1 tsp. of Xanthan gum
- ¾ tsp. of baking powder
- ¾ tsp. of baking soda
- ¼ tsp. of salt

- 1 tbsp. of poppy seed
- 2 scoops of low carb protein powder (the Jamie Eason lean body protein powder is preferred).

Directions:

1. Pre-heat your oven to about 350 degrees F, and then coat lightly, 8 muffin cups (standard sizes), with a non-stick cooking spray.
2. Get a medium to large bowl, and inside whisk together, the coconut flour, alongside Xanthan gum, baking powder, salt, baking soda, poppy seeds, and lemon zest, and stir properly to ensure adequate mixing.
3. Get a separate bowl and inside whisk together the coconut oil or butter with the vanilla, before mixing in the yogurt until there are no large lumps remaining.
4. Stir in the agave, alongside the almond milk, and lemon juice, then mixes the protein powder into the mix.

5. Add the coconut flour mix, then stir the entire mix until they are perfectly blended.
6. Let the batter sit for about 10 minutes.
7. Divide your dough in-between your prepared muffin cups, and then bake them for about 24 minutes inside the 350 degrees F oven, and insert a toothpick after baking, if it comes out clean then the muffins are done.
8. Cool the muffins in a pan for about 5 minutes before you turn them out into the wire rack.

Eggplant Mozzarella Casserole

Ingredients:

- 3/4 cup almond flour, 3 ounces
- 3/4 cup grated parmesan cheese, 3 ounces
- 1/2 teaspoon garlic powder
- 1/2 teaspoon Italian seasoning
- Salt and pepper, to taste
- 1 eggplant, about 1 1/4 pounds before trimming
- 8 ounces mozzarella cheese, shredded
- Breading mixture:
- 2 eggs
- Nonstick cooking spray

Directions:
To make breading:

1. Combine all of the dry Ingredients: in a pie pan.
2. Break the eggs into a cereal bowl and beat well with a fork.
3. Position your oven rack in the center position. Preheat the broiler to 500F°.
4. Cut the eggplant into twelve slices of even thickness.
5. Dip each piece of eggplant in egg to coat on both sides, then lightly coat them with parmesan-almond mixture.
6. Arrange the eggplant slices on a foil-lined baking sheet in a single layer.
7. Spray the eggplant liberally with cooking spray.
8. Broil about 3 minutes until golden brown; turn over, spray again with cooking spray and broil the other side. Watch it closely to prevent burning.
9. Spray an 8x8" baking pan with cooking spray.

10. Arrange a layer of eggplant over the bottom of the pan, cutting them to fill the gaps.
11. Sprinkle half of the shredded cheese over the eggplant.
12. Repeat layering eggplant and cheese.
13. Bake at 350F° about 20-30 minutes until the cheese is bubbly and golden brown on top.
14. Cut into squares and serve with tomato sauce, if desired.

Green Chile Frittata

Ingredients:

- 1 (7 ounce) can diced green chile peppers, drained
- 1 (16 ounce) container cottage cheese
- 1 cup shredded cheddar cheese
- 1/4 cup melted butter
- 10 eggs, beaten
- 1/2 cup coconut flour
- 1 teaspoon baking powder
- 1 pinch salt

Directions:

1. Preheat oven to 400 F. Lightly grease a 9x13 inch baking dish.
2. In a large bowl, mix the eggs, flour, baking powder, and salt.

3. Stir in the green chile peppers, cottage cheese, cheddar cheese, and melted butter. Pour into the prepared baking dish.
4. Bake 15 minutes in the preheated oven. Reduce heat to 325 F, and continue baking for 35 to 40 minutes.
5. Cool slightly, and cut into small squares.

Crisp Meringue Cookies

Ingredients:

- 1/4 teaspoon of cream of tartar
- 6 tablespoons of swerve confectioners pinch of salt
- 4 large egg whites
- 1/2 teaspoon of almond extract

Directions:

1. Preheat your broiler to 210 degrees. Empty your egg whites into your blending bowl, then, at that point, add your cream of tartar.
2. Start your blender gradually and increment towards a medium speed.
3. At the point when your egg whites begin to look foamy stop the blender and add 3 tablespoons of Swerve, the almond extricate, and salt.

4. Mix on a rapid until your egg whites prepare to a medium consistency.
5. Stop your blender and add the leftover 3 tablespoons of Swerve.
6. Continue to whip on a fast until your meringue turns out to be extremely solid and begins to pull away from the sides of the bowl.
7. Stop the mixer and scrape the meringue out of the whisk and down the sides of the bowl, then mix it again to make sure that everything is mixed evenly.
8. Load your meringue into a funneling sack fitted with a huge star-molded tip.
9. Contingent upon the size of your sack you might have to top off the pack a couple of times to deal with the whole batch.
10. Place sheets of material paper on 2 to 3 baking sheets.

11. The number of you want will rely upon how intently you can easily pipe the treats close to one another.
12. Pipe out 18 rosette shapes, or whatever shape you prefer.
13. Bake your meringue treats for around 40 minutes at 210 degrees.
14. Whenever they are done switch the broiler off and air out the entryway, then, at that point, permit them to cool for another 30 minutes.

Double Chocolate Bundt Cake

Ingredients:

white chocolate glaze:

- 2 tablespoons of Heavy Cream
- 3 tablespoons of Powdered Erythritol
- 1 teaspoon of Vanilla Extract
- 2 ounces of Anthony's Organic Cocoa Butter

Wafers bundt cake:

- 3 Large Eggs
- 2 cups of Anthony's Almond Flour
- 1 cup of Butter
- 1 1/2 teaspoons of Baking Soda
- 2 tablespoons of Coconut Flour
- 1/2 cup of Sour Cream
- 1 cup of Erythritol
- 1 cup of Water

- 1/2 teaspoon of Salt
- 2 teaspoons of Vanilla Extract
- 1/2 cup of Cocoa Powder

Directions:

1. Preheat your stove to 350 degrees.
2. Whisk together 2 cups of Anthony's Blanched Almond Flour with your baking pop, salt, coconut flour, and erythritol.
3. Heat up your margarine, water, and cocoa powder in a little pot over medium hotness. Rush until it is consolidated and afterward take off heat.
4. Pour a large portion of your chocolate blend into your dry blend and mix it to join. When it thickens, pour in other half and mix to consolidate again.
5. Add 1 egg at a time to your mixture.
6. Add your vanilla concentrate and sharp cream. Mix well.

7. Pour your blend into a lubed bundt cake dish. Heat roughly 40 to 50 minutes.
8. Prepare glaze while cake prepares. Dissolve your cocoa spread wafers.
9. Add powdered erythritol and mix to consolidate.
10. Add weighty cream and spot in cooler. Take out and mix around each 5 minutes.
11. Once murky and thick, mix in blender until it is smooth.
12. Once your cake is finished heating up, permit it to cool in its prospect 10 minutes.
13. Transform onto a cooling rack on your baking sheet or plate. Permit it to totally cool.
14. Glaze your cake. While your frosting is wet, sprinkle your cocoa nibs over your cake. Permit the coating to chill off and harden.

Fried egg with ham and broccoli

Ingredients:

- 15g dill
- 2 eggs size m
- Some olive oil
- 50g cooked ham
- 50g broccoli
- Sea salt and pepper

Directions:

1. First cut the boiled ham into cubes and then wash the broccoli. Depending on the size and taste, chop the individual broccoli florets.
2. Then wash the dill, shake dry and finely chop.
3. Heat the olive oil in a pan and fry the broccoli in it.
4. Then beat the eggs into the pan and generously sprinkle the dill over it.

5. Add the diced ham and finish frying the eggs over medium heat.
6. Season the finished fried eggs with pepper and sea salt and drizzle with a little olive oil.

Rocket and tomato salad with mozzarella

Ingredients:

- 10g chia seeds
- Some olive oil
- Some balsamic vinegar
- Sea salt and pepper
- 100g cherry tomatoes
- 100g rocket
- 50g mozzarella
- 25g walnut kernels

Directions:

1. Wash the rocket, shake dry and cut off the long stalks.
2. Wash the cherry tomatoes and cut in half. Then cut the mozzarella into thin slices.

3. Now mix the rocket, the halved cherry tomatoes, the mozzarella and the walnuts in a bowl.
4. Sprinkle the salad with chia seeds and season with sea salt and pepper.
5. Finally, add some balsamic vinegar and olive oil.

Coconut Oil-Fried Eggs and Vegetables

Ingredients:

- Eggs (3 or 4)
- Spices
- Optional: Spinach
- Coconut oil
- Frozen Vegetable Mix – green beans, broccoli, cauliflower, carrots

Directions:

1. Heat a frying pan and put in the coconut oil.
2. When the oil is hot enough, put in the vegetable mix. Let the frozen vegetables thaw in the heat.
3. Add eggs.
4. Add spices according to your tastes.
5. Add the spinach.
6. Stir fry until cooked to your preferences.

Mexican Veal Sausages

Ingredients:

- ½ teaspoon of salt
- ½ teaspoon of ground cumin
- 2 tablespoons of green or red salsa
- 2 tablespoons of fresh cilantro, chopped
- 2 green onions, finely chopped, 1/3 cup
- 1 ½ pounds ground veal
- 1 lime, cut into slices for garnish
- ¼ cup of sour cream for garnish
- ¼ cup of green or red salsa for garnish
- 2 tablespoons of olive oil
- ¼ teaspoon freshly ground pepper

Directions:

1. Onion, veal and all spices should be combined in a large mixing bowl and blended together

2. Mixture should then be shaped into 4 sausage links
3. Oil should be heated in a non-stick skillet on high heat and brown sausage to about 8 to 10 minutes, turning should be frequently done

Carolina Style Barbeque Meatballs

Ingredients:

For the meatballs

- ¼ teaspoon cayenne pepper
- ¼ teaspoon ground cumin
- ¼ teaspoon celery salt
- ¼ egg
- 2 tablespoons almond flour
- ½ tablespoon water
- ¼ lb. ground pork
- ¼ teaspoon granulated sugar substitute (honey for Paleo)
- ¼ teaspoon paprika (smoked if you have it)
- ¼ teaspoon salt
- ¼ teaspoon black pepper

For the low carb BBQ sauce

- 1 tablespoon honey
- ¼ tablespoon apple cider vinegar
- ¼ tablespoon low sugar ketchup
- Salt, to taste
- 2 tablespoons yellow mustard
- ½ teaspoon Hot Sauce
- ¼ tablespoon dried onion flakes
- Pepper, to taste

Directions:

For the low carb BBQ sauce

1. Place all the Ingredients: of the sauce in a small saucepan and mix well until well combined.
2. Heat over a low flame for about 8 minutes until simmering.

For the meatballs

3. Combine all the Ingredients: for the meatballs in a medium sized mixing bowl until well combined. Divide the meatball mix into 4 equal parts and form into smooth balls.
4. Heat a little oil in a large non-stick frying pan and lightly fry the meatballs until well browned and cooked through. It should take about 4 minutes per side to cook.
5. Douse the meatballs in the prepared barbeque sauce and spread the sauce and meatballs onto a parchment lined baking sheet. Broil for about 3 to 4 minutes.
6. Serve hot with some low carb coleslaw.
7. Enjoy!

Cheese Enchiladas

Ingredients:

For the Enchiladas

- 2 eggs, well beaten
- 1 ½ cups mozzarella, grated
- 1 ½ cups frozen cauliflower, thawed, drained and processed / diced

For the Enchilada Sauce

- 1 teaspoon cumin
- ½ teaspoon salt
- 1/4 teaspoon pepper
- ½ cup pizza sauce or low sugar tomato sauce
- 1 cup cheddar cheese, shredded
- 1 cup monterey jack or pepper jack, shredded
- ¼ Cup onion, chopped
- 1 large clove of garlic, chopped or crushed

- ½ tablespoon chili powder

- 2 tablespoons extra virgin olive oil

- ½ teaspoon oregano

Directions:

For the Enchiladas

1. Crank up the oven to 450 degrees F and allow the oven to preheat.
2. Combine the processed cauliflower, grated cheese and eggs together in a mixing bowl.
3. Grease a cookie sheet and pour about 1/3 cup of the dough into 6, 6-inch rounds.
4. Place the cookie sheet into the preheated oven and bake for about 15 minutes or until the edges of the shell brown and the whole crust has a golden hue to it.
5. Remove the shells from the oven and cool the shells before loosening the shells from the pan.
6. Once the shell is set, place the shell aside.

For the Enchilada Sauce

1. Crank up the oven to 350 degrees F and allow the oven to preheat.
2. Pour the oil into a saucepan and heat on a medium high flame until lightly smoking.
3. Add the garlic, onion and chili powder to it and sauté for about 5 minutes or until tender.
4. Add in the oregano, salt, pizza sauce, cumin, and pepper to the pan and mix well.
5. Keep mixing until the sauce is heated through.
6. Add in about half the cheeses and mix well.
7. Take the prepared shells and dip into the heated enchilada sauce.
8. Place the sauce dipped shells, golden size up, onto an ungreased 9 x 13 inch casserole dish.
9. Spoon about 2 tablespoons of the remaining cheeses into the shells and roll into a tight roll.
10. Place the enchiladas, seam side down and top with the remaining enchilada sauce.

11. Pop into the oven and bake for about 20 to 25 minutes until the cheese is gooey and bubbly.
12. Serve immediately.
13. Enjoy!

Swedish Meatballs

Ingredients:

- 1 small egg
- Salt, to taste
- 2 tablespoons seasoned breadcrumbs
- Pepper, to taste
- 1 cup reduced sodium beef stock
- ¼ teaspoon allspice
- 1 oz. light cream cheese
- ½ teaspoon olive oil
- 1 clove garlic, minced
- ½ small onion, minced
- ½ celery stalk, minced
- ½ lb. 93% lean ground beef
- 2 tablespoons minced parsley

Directions:

1. Pour the oil into a deep sauté pan and heat over a medium high flame. Add in the onion and garlic and sauté until the garlic is aromatic and the onion is translucent. This should take about 5 minutes.
2. Add in the parsley and celery and cook for another 4 to 5 minutes, or until tender. Allow the sautéed vegetables to cool slightly.
3. Combine the beef, sautéed vegetable mixture, salt, allspice, egg, breadcrumbs and pepper together in a large mixing bowl. Mix well.
4. Scoop out about 2 tablespoons of the meatball mix and form into a smooth meatball.
5. Pour the beef stock into a pan and heat on a high flame until bubbling. Reduce the heat to a medium low and slowly put the meatballs into the pan.

6. Cover the pan with a lid and cook for about 20 minutes.
7. Using a slotted spoon, drain the meatballs from the broth and place on a serving dish.
8. Strain the stock and pour into a blender jar. Add in the cream cheese and pulse until it forms a smooth mix.
9. Return the broth and cream cheese mix into the pan and simmer the sauce until it thickens.
10. Pour the sauce over the prepared meatballs and serve immediately with toothpicks or over some gluten free noodles.
11. Enjoy!

Russian Stir-Fry

Ingredients:

- 1 c mushrooms
- 1 c spinach
- 200g bubbled sweet potato
- 200g chicken bosom, cubed
- 1 tbsp. of bean stew garlic sauce
- 2 huge cabbage leaves

Directions:

1. Brown the chicken in a skillet showered with Pam on medium heat.
2. Once the chicken is mostly cooked, add the remainder of the Ingredients:.
3. Cover and cook for 5-7 minutes on high. 4. Plate and enjoy!

Chicken Breast Mushroom Sandwich

Ingredients:

- 2 cuts of 4:9 Ezekiel bread
- Salt and pepper (to taste)
- Dijon mustard
- Calorie free hot sauce
- 1 c of cut mushrooms
- 1 tail of green onions, sliced
- 100g chicken bosom, cut on a level plane into a cutlet

Directions:
1. Toast the Ezekiel bread.
2. In a dish showered with Pam, sauté mushrooms and onions with pepper and salt.
3. Once the vegetables are prepared, remove them from the container and put aside.

4. Spray the skillet with Pam and cook the chicken bosom, adding salt and pepper.
5. For the chicken bosom is getting singed, sprinkle a few hot sauce on one cut of toast and mustard on the other.
6. On the toast sprinkled with hot sauce, mount the vegetables.
7. Once the chicken is prepared, set it on top of the vegetables and finish it off with the other piece of toast.

Strawberry Greek Yogurt Whip

Ingredients:

- Frozen strawberries 3
- Low-fat milk ½ cup
- Light whipped topping ½ cup
- No-cal sweetener 1 tbs
- Fat-free Greek yogurt ⅔ cup

Directions:

1. Add the strawberries to a bowl and allow them to defrost.
2. Dice up the strawberries until they are well chopped and slightly runny. Blend with Greek yogurt and milk.
3. Add in the sweetener and mix well.
4. Fold the whipped topping into the mixture.
5. Enjoy this immediately or cover and refrigerate it until later.

Winter Sunshine Smoothie

Ingredients:

- Unsweetened coconut milk, 2 tbs
- Chilled unsweetened coconut water, 1 cup
- Rolled porridge oats, ⅓ cup
- Fresh ginger ½ inch piece
- Fresh turmeric ½ inch piece
- Segmented and peeled Clementine 2

Directions:

1. Add the oats to a blender and pulse until it turns into a finely ground powder.
2. Add in the ginger, turmeric, Clementine, coconut milk, and coconut water and pulse until they come together.
3. Pour your smoothie into a glass and enjoy.

www.ingramcontent.com/pod-product-compliance
Lightning Source LLC
Chambersburg PA
CBHW050244120526
44590CB00016B/2212